BEE H

THORSONS NUTRIENTS FOR HEALTH

BEE HEALTH

——

HASNAIN WALJI, PH.D.

Thorsons
An Imprint of HarperCollinsPublishers

Thorsons
An Imprint of HarperCollins*Publishers*
77–85 Fulham Palace Road
Hammersmith, London W6 8JB

1160 Battery Street
San Francisco, California 94111–1213

Published by Thorsons 1996
1 3 5 7 9 10 8 6 4 2

A catalogue record for this book
is available from the British Library

ISBN 0 7225 3323 3

Printed and bound in Great Britain by
Caledonian International Book Manufacturing Ltd, Glasgow

To the seekers of health and to those
who help them find it naturally.

Contents

Acknowledgements

I would like to express my deep gratitude to David Ponsonby and Auriel Mott for assisting me with the research. I also wish to thank my wife, Latifa, for her patience and endurance as I devoted time to my research, not to mention her gentle care and concern, which enabled me to complete this book.

Preface

The bee is more honoured than other animals, not because she labours, but because she labours for others.

John Chrysostom (AD 383)

Some time ago, a British tabloid revealed that Britain's Royal Family supplemented their diets with royal jelly and bee pollen. The story was further sensationalized by the allegation, from an inside source, that Princess Diana took these bee products at Prince Charles' insistence.

Whatever the truth of the matter, British Royalty is by no means unique, nor the first, to recognize the benefits of bee products. Since antiquity, royals and their subjects have used these products of the hive for improving health and vitality. So, what is it that makes bee products so helpful in our efforts to attain health and wellbeing?

Like bee pollen, which is said to be worth its weight in gold, all bee products are packed with nutrients – amino acids, minerals, vitamins, enzymes and coenzymes – required for good health. This is their strength, for the following reasons. When we think about supplementing our diets, it is tempting to think in terms of taking just one particular vitamin or group of vitamins. However, it has been found that vitamins and minerals work best when they are taken, not singly, but in conjunction with others. The actions of some enhance the actions of others, so there is less likely to be an imbalance if they are taken together. This is where bee products come into their own as they contain a number of enzymes, vitamins, minerals, amino acids, carbohydrates and hormones that work together to promote health. Bee products fit perfectly into the 'food as medicine' category (the basis of nutritional therapy) and have been around for thousands of years – they have stood the test of time. This book, based on the findings of many scientists and researchers, is written to help you learn more about these healing foods.

During my research for this book, one study summed up the special quality of bee products. Professor Nicolai Vasilievich Tsitsin, a researcher at the Longevity Institute of Russia, sought to find the main reason so many natives of Georgia (Russia) were living up to and beyond 100 years. It turned out that a majority of these centenarians were beekeepers. As part of their daily diet they ate raw, unprocessed honey with bee pollen!

Of late it is propolis which has been the focus of attention in our quest for natural substances that protect us from the ravages of infections and help boost our immune system. It is this gem from the treasures of the hive that is being hailed as an effective natural antibiotic, which can help us fight a whole host of ailments, from a sore throat to radiation injury.

Hasnain Walji
Milton Keynes
May 1996

1

Did You Know ... ?

Most of us don't give insects a second thought unless we happen to be stung by one or they inconvenience us in other ways. We are even less likely to think that they may actually be of some benefit to us. Perhaps the bee is the one exception. We all know about honey. Indeed, many of us regularly consume it as part of our daily diet, as a sweetener in cooking or as a spread on our sandwiches or toast. We are even vaguely aware that it has some medicinal properties and can be a soothing balm for sore throats when we come down with a cold.

Honey is not the only substance bees manufacture that has been found to have benefits for humankind. There are also bee pollen, beeswax, royal jelly, propolis and even bee venom. That such a variety of products can come from such small creatures can be best explained if we look at the life of the bee and how its society is organized.

As we all know, bees live in hives. Hives are comprised of rows of eight-sided cells, which we know better as honeycomb. These cells are made out of beeswax, which the bees, having consumed large quantities of honey, manufacture inside glands in their abdomen and then chew to soften, ready to be moulded into shape. They use 'bee glue', or propolis, to attach the honeycomb to the hive and to repair cracks or fill in spaces and even disinfect the hive. Pollen is gathered by bees as food for their young and it has been shown that, for a colony of bees to survive, it must have between 22.5 and 32 kg (50 and 70 lbs) of pollen. Royal jelly is a special food secreted by the worker bees and fed, initially, to all the larvae, but, after three days, exclusively to the future queen bee. Bee venom is the poison released in the sting of a bee.

There are thousands of bees in a hive. Some authorities put the figure at between 40,000 and 60,000, others at between 25,000 and 100,000. Each bee has its own task in the hive. Although there are just three types of bee, there is only one queen – the rest are either workers or drones, with workers greatly outnumbering the drones.

The role of the queen is to lay eggs, perhaps as many as 2,000 a day. She is fertilized by the drones, these male bees dying once they have mated with her. If she is not fertilized, the queen will continue to lay eggs, but they will hatch out as drones. If she is fertilized, then the larvae will be females and it is the females who are the workers. Worker bees are charged with the responsibility of building and maintaining the hive, gathering the nectar from which to make honey and collecting the pollen, feeding and rearing the queen bee's young, fanning the hive with their wings and protecting the hive against outside marauders.

Worker bees live only for a season, but, in the wild, the queen bee may survive for as long as five or six years. In hives which are kept for the continuous production of honey and other bee products, the process of 'requeening' a hive is performed by the beekeeper who, each year, removes an ageing queen and substitutes a younger and more virile queen.

Worker bees are anatomically different from the queen bee, even though they are all female. The worker bee has a larger brain than the queen. Her hind legs have combs for collecting the pollen, which is brushed onto her body as she enters a flower looking for nectar. These legs also have a press for compacting the pollen and baskets in which to store it. Her mouth is so constructed as to be able to suck the nectar from the flower, chew pollen, propolis and wax and attack enemies.

The queen has none of these attributes and cannot even feed herself, relying entirely on the workers to perform that function for her. However, she has the reproductive equipment to lay thousands of eggs. She deposits the eggs through an ovipositor and has a sperm storage sac in her abdomen. A queen is made, however, and not born. Eggs destined to become workers are deposited in cells about 0.5 cm (¼ in) across. The cell for the future queen is a different shape altogether and is larger. Scientific observation has discovered that any female larva under four days old placed in the queen cell will turn into a queen. However, it is not the size of the cell that determines whether its inhabitant develops into a queen. What the cell does is to act as a sort of marker, distinguishing it from the other cells so that the workers continue to feed the larva within it the royal jelly that, on the fourth day, is withdrawn from the other larvae. The rest of the grubs go on to become mere worker bees.

The layout of the hive is ordered so that the brood cells are located near the centre of the comb. The cells containing the honey and the bee pollen surround the brood cells. Honey cells have a thin covering of wax. With human intervention, the construction of a hive is more controlled, although modern hives try to replicate the natural order. Old-fashioned hives might have been made from roughly hewn logs or from clay shaped into a cylinder or have taken the form of woven, conical straw baskets. With the discovery that bees need spaces of between 1 and 1.3 cm (⅜ to ½ in) in which to pass through the hive, that they could be 'trained' to make straight rows of honeycomb by being given a sheet of beeswax imprinted with the hexagonal shapes of the cells and with the introduction of the use of centrifugal force to separate the liquid honey from the wax, the modern hive was developed with its removable top and frames. In these hives, the young bees are reared in the lower level and honey and bee pollen are kept in the upper levels. This layout makes it easy for the beekeeper to remove the upper frames containing the honey while leaving the rest of the bee colony alone.

Honey

Honey starts out as nectar in flowers. The bee sucks out the nectar through its long, tube-like tongue. The sweet liquid is then stored in the bee's honey gland or sac and mixes with certain chemicals in the gland. When the bee returns to the hive, the nectar and chemical mixture is deposited in the cells where it then ripens to become honey. Bees are selective about the flowers from which they draw nectar and may travel up to 2 miles to find just the right flower. They are attracted by colour as well as fragrance, with yellow and blue flowers being preferred.

Just as there are hundreds of different varieties of flower, so there are just as many varieties of honey, and each will also be affected by the weather and climate in which the plant grows, the quality of the soil, how ripe the honey was when harvested and how the honey was subsequently processed. Honey is comprised of highly concentrated sugars, with vitamins, minerals, pollen grains, water and enzymes featuring as well.

Does honey have anything to offer modern humankind beyond being a sweetening agent?

In the United States alone, some 12,500 tons of honey is

harvested annually. Most of it is used for sweetening and, indeed, it has been found to be a source of quick energy. It has preservative properties as well, however, and has been used as an antiseptic and an antibiotic. In fact, it is surprisingly versatile and its uses are diverse, ranging from cuts and bruises, chapped skin, constipation, diarrhoea, sore throats, warts, facial treatments and hand lotions to curing pipe bowls, chewing gum, spray adhesive, centres of golf balls, antifreeze, baby food and to treat malnutrition, rickets, scurvy, anaemia, intestinal disorders and wounds.

Beeswax

Beeswax is the building material from which the hive is constructed and which seals off the honey cells. The bee ingests large amounts of honey from which the wax is manufactured in one of the glands, or stomachs, of the bee. The wax is made into flakes that are then moulded by the bee into the desired shape.

We have found a large number of uses for beeswax, including cosmetics, candles, chewing gum, medical ointments and pill coatings, to name just a few.

Propolis

This substance is derived from the sweet-smelling resin that is exuded by the leaf buds and bark of trees, especially poplars and conifers, to deter pests. The bee collects the resin by biting off a piece and chewing it to soften it before transferring it into the pollen baskets on her back legs. Once the bee returns to the hive, she waits for other bees to remove what they need to use for their work. The process of removal may take up to several hours.

Collection of resin is not a continuous process. Indeed,

it only takes place at particular times of the year – mainly in August, September and October – and on the sunniest days when it is at its softest and so is easiest to break off.

Propolis has two main uses. First, as it has disinfective properties, it helps to protect the colony from bacterial and viral infections. In fact, before the queen even lays an egg, the cell is cleaned out by the workers and lined with a very fine coating of propolis so that the environment for the hatching larva is a sterile one.

Second, because it has glue-like characteristics, it is used to fix loose bits of the hive that might become damaged by cold and rain. The bees also construct complicated entrances to the hive so that not many bees are needed to police bees and other insects going into the hive. Intruders that are successful in gaining entry and which are stung to death, are wrapped around with propolis and then embalmed with wax so that infection that would otherwise be caused by the dead animal decaying is prevented. The surface of the hive is itself coated with propolis and then polished by the bees to ensure that their wings are not damaged by any rough edges.

Propolis has been analysed and has been found to be comprised of 50 to 55 per cent resins and balsams, 30 per cent beeswax, 10 to 15 per cent essential oils and 5 per cent bee pollen. The most active part of the resins are bioflavonoids, which are able to control micro-organisms and help to stimulate the immune system in humans.

Bee Pollen

Earlier it was mentioned that bees collect pollen for feeding to their young, but pollen is, of course, part of the plant world's reproductive process. In fact, pollen is the male seed, which must fertilize the female parts of the plant. The spread of pollen is carried out either by the wind (the types of pollen spread this way are light) or by insects, mainly bees, as they enter the plant to gather nectar and pollen (these are heavier). It is the light varieties of pollen that are responsible for the unpleasant effects of hayfever. Heavier pollens are never airborne and so do not cause a problem.

If the purpose of a bee's visit to a plant is to gather pollen, she mixes saliva and nectar with the pollen grains and packs them in her pollen baskets on her back legs. When she visits another flower, the pollen from the previous one that she has picked up on the hairs of her body are brushed off, thereby pollinating the next flower and so on. More than 80 per cent of plants are pollinated in this way by the bee and it has been calculated that if the bee did not perform this useful function, in excess of 100,000 plant species would become extinct.

It is possible for a bee to collect 4,000,000 grains of pollen in one hour, visiting around 1,000 different flowers in the process.

Royal Jelly

Also known as 'bee milk', this secretion is manufactured from pollen in the third gland located in the worker bee and it changes a female grub from a potential worker into the queen bee. All larvae are fed with royal jelly for the first three days of their lives, but then it is withdrawn from the others and fed only to the queen. Throughout the queen's life and wherever she goes, she is licked by the worker bees. The royal jelly is passed from their tongues onto her body and then absorbed. The other bees are sustained by a mixture of pollen, nectar and water.

Not only does the queen live considerably longer than other bees, she is also almost twice as big and is highly fertile, whereas the workers are infertile. The queen reaches sexual maturity after only 16 days whereas it takes 21 days for the workers to mature. The queen starts laying her numerous eggs from day 16 and it is royal jelly that keeps her so productive.

Bee Venom

It is obvious what use a bee sting is to the insect itself, although, sadly, for a worker bee it can only use its stinger once. It then dies. The queen bee, on the other hand, has a differently shaped stinger and she is able to use it several times over – not in protecting the hive, but in the destruction of a rival queen bee or other queen larvae that have not yet emerged. There can be only one queen in a hive. Strange as it may seem, the sting of the bee has been found to have benefits for humans, which beekeepers, among others, can testify to.

This is, perhaps, the most controversial of the bee products, particularly as bee stings can sometimes cause an adverse, if not fatal, reaction in certain people. However, it is an interesting fact that bee stings have been found to have produced dramatic beneficial results in the treatment of arthritis. The components of bee venom credited with these effects are mellitin and apamin, as well as an enzyme that is able to identify rheumatoid molecules in the lubricating fluid between the joints. Further research in Russia has revealed that the venom stimulates the production of cortisone, a natural anti-inflammatory.

The Products of the Hive in History

Bees have existed for much longer than we humans. The American Museum of History in New York holds what is probably the oldest known bee, preserved in a piece of fossilized amber. The amber is thought to be around

80,000,000 years old, but the bee trapped inside it may be even older.

A cave painting found near Valencia in Spain, dating back to the Mesolithic era, depicts a human figure perched on a ladder removing honey from a hive and fighting off the bees. This cave is known as Cueva de la Arana, the Cave of the Spiders.

Honey has been a part of humankind's culinary and medicinal repertoire perhaps as far back as prehistoric times, as has been discovered by archaeologists. The use of honey and its associated products has been found to date back to the major ancient civilizations and, perhaps, earlier.

The ancient Egyptians were certainly aware of their properties. Indeed, they revered the bee and often used it as a motif in their ornaments and on official documents. They would offer honey and pollen to the gods and supplies were left for the dead as food in the afterlife. They would make gifts of honey to those whose esteem they sought and, at weddings, the bridegroom was required to give honey to the bride. The pharaohs extolled the virtues of bees, citing them as a model of hard work and total devotion to their queen.

Honey, bee pollen and propolis were used in their medicines and surgical dressings. Honey and bee pollen were taken internally to cure ulcers, act as a laxative and combat worms. Eye infections were also treated with these substances.

The ancient Greeks were equally devoted to the bee and her wares. Hippocrates (460–377BC), the 'father of modern medicine', used propolis in his treatments. Indeed, he used honey daily, stating that, 'It causes heat, cleans sores and ulcers, softens hard ulcers of the lips, heals carbuncles and running sores'.

He wasn't the only influential Greek to extol the virtues of honey as many of his contemporaries experimented with honey diets. Democritus, who is said to have solved the 'riddle of the atom and matter', consumed a diet rich in honey and finally died at the age of 109. Pythagoras and his disciples were also keen consumers, as were poets, philosophers, writers and other academics – all believing that honey was capable of extending lifespan and curing many ills. Honey and bee pollen were taken liberally by the Olympic athletes in their daily diets and, just before an event, they would imbibe a honey and water drink to give them energy and stamina.

Even the Greek gods succumbed to the influence of the humble bee. Ambrosia – a concoction of milk and honey – was believed to be the elixir that preserved their immortality. Aphrodite, the goddess of love, fed honey to her consorts. Greek honey was famed for its curative powers, especially the honey from Attica and Mount Hymettus.

What was good for the Greeks was also good for the Romans. The Roman scholar Pliny wrote extensively about the nutritional and medicinal benefits of honey, bee pollen and propolis. Of propolis he commented how it 'extracts stings and all substances embedded in the flesh, reduces swelling, softens hardened areas, soothes pain of the sinews and heals sores when it appears hopeless for them to mend'.

Other civilizations and other times have placed great store by the beneficial actions of bee products. In ancient times, Britain was known as 'the Honey Isle of Beli' because of the large amounts of honey harvested.

In China, bee pollen was the more highly regarded bee product, being collected in special nets floated on lakes. A poultice of honey and bee pollen was applied to irritated skin sores. The Maoris of New Zealand made cakes out of cat's tail pollen and Apache and Pueblo Indians used the same pollen and maize in their fertility rituals.

In a chapter entitled 'the Bee', The Koran proclaims, 'From out of their bellies comes a drink of different colours in which there is healing for mankind'. The Prophet Mohammed is believed to have said that 'honey is a remedy for all diseases'.

The Rig-Veda, written in Sanskrit between 2000 and 3000BC, a holy book of the Hindus, mentions bees with reverence and Vishnu, one of the Hindu trinity of gods, is frequently depicted as a blue bee on a lotus flower.

In more recent times, John Gerard, the herbalist, referred in his herbal *The Historie of Plants*, in 1597, to the healing powers of propolis and Nicholas Culpeper stated in his famous work that 'the ointment called propolis is singularly good for all heat and inflammations in any part of the body, and tempers the heat of wounds'.

During the Boer War (1899–1902), wounds were treated with propolis and petroleum jelly, with dried moss as dressings.

In Roman mythology, Jupiter transformed Melissa into a bee so that she could prepare the healing substance propolis.

It is hoped that, in some way, the attributes of bee products will transform your life, too – for the better.

2

Bee Pollen: The Most Complete Food

How can such tiny things as pollen have any beneficial influences on human beings? After all, they are so small (50/1000ths of a millimetre) that it takes over 14,000 of the largest to weigh 1 g (less than $\frac{1}{16}$ oz). You would need 8,000,000 pollen grains from the spruce tree to make up 25 g (1 oz) in weight. However, scientists are recognizing that the body needs more than just the basic, well-known nutrients for the body to function well. The body also requires what are known as micronutrients, which bee pollen has been found to contain. In fact, medical trials are now validating what many have known all along.

In 1961, in a paper presented by Robert Delperee entitled 'The Secrets of the Life of Bees', it was demonstrated by reference to chemical analyses of bee pollen in laboratories around the world that bee pollen has the nutritional capacity to sustain life. In 1963, the Lee Foundation for Nutritional Research of Milwaukee reported that bee pollen is so perfectly balanced that it could stand on its own as a complete food, provided it was augmented with roughage and water.

No complete analysis has been made of bee pollen as it is so complex. Nevertheless, we do know that it contains vitamins, minerals, amino acids (the building blocks of proteins), enzymes and fatty acids.

In the past, honey and bee pollen together have been used to treat disorders ranging from bowel irregularity to kidney diseases, respiratory difficulties and skin irritations, even for more severe cases, such as burns. It has also been used as a relaxant and as an aphrodisiac. In modern times, bee pollen has been found to help in such conditions as allergies, digestion and prostate disorders, in reducing the distressing effects of chemotherapy and in improving athletic performance. Cosmetics, too, may contain bee pollen.

Apart from the nutritional and therapeutic benefits of bee pollen, its other main advantage is that it is easily digested and taken up by the body. Indeed, it has been shown to act quickly because it does not have to go through the normal processes of digestion and can actually be absorbed direct from the stomach into the bloodstream. After only 30 minutes, bee pollen grains can be found in the blood, their structure having undergone substantial alteration in the meantime. This transference from the stomach to the bloodstream is known as persorption. In a study on dogs fed on bee pollen in milk cream, whole grains were found in their blood, urine and cerebral spinal fluids two hours later. Similar results have been observed in humans (Jorde and Linskens, 1974).

A Complete Food

Bee pollen has been found to contain all the nutrients known to man. It is, as mentioned earlier, a complete food. The average composition of bee pollen is 60 per cent carbohydrates, 20 per cent protein, 7 per cent fat, 7 per cent water and 6 per cent minerals, but, of course, the actual content depends on the particular type of pollen, the quality of the soil in which the plant is grown, the location and climate.

As far as the protein content is concerned, bee pollen

contains all the known amino acids. Bees need to obtain eight of these from their diets, as do humans. These are, isoleucine, leucine, lysine, methionine, phenylalanine, thereonine, tryptophan and valine. A further two, arginine and histidine, are what Leon Chaitow, a naturopathic practitioner and writer specializing in alternative health, calls 'of ambiguous state' (*Amino Acids in Therapy*) and may be required during different phases of life. Tests have revealed that bee pollen is a balanced source of all the essential amino acids.

Comparisons have been made between the protein content of bee pollen and that of other foods. It has been found that bee pollen is a 'superior source' of amino acids compared to whole egg and cow's milk, and it contains more lysine, leucine and glutamic acid than do either of these foods.

Research has also been carried out to see whether or not pollen collected by bees varies nutritionally from pollen collected by hand. In other words, is there anything special about bee pollen? In fact, pollen collected by bees has been proved to be nutritionally better than hand-collected pollen.

One study looked at the protein content of hand-gathered pollens from desert plants and compared it with the protein content of pollen collected from citrus flowers. It was found that the protein content of the desert plants ranged from 7 to 15.6 per cent, whereas for the citrus flowers the range was between 6.2 and 20.7 per cent. However, when a further comparison was made between these and pollen gathered by honey bees, the protein content of the pollen gathered by bees was found to be between 17.1 and 22.6 per cent (Gilliam, McCaughey and B. Wintermute, 1980).

The carbohydrate and fat content of pollen varies from plant to plant. Conifer pollen, for example, is lower in carbohydrates than that from flowering plants. Fructose, glucose and sucrose are the main natural sugars in pollen.

The fibre content averages out at just under 8 per cent.

Fats make up an average of about 5 per cent and the three main fatty acids are arachidonic, linoleic and linolenic acids. These three fatty acids (known as essential fatty acids) provide the material for the formation of prostaglandins (hormone-like substances), which have the ability to control inflammation, regulate blood pressure, body temperature and affect the action of other hormones in the body.

As for minerals, pollen contains potassium, phosphorous, sulphur, calcium, selenium, sodium, magnesium, iron, aluminium, copper, manganese, nickel, titanium, zinc, chlorine, silicon, boron, iodine, barium, strontium and molybdenum.

Dr Lunden, who has done considerable research on pollen, has found that pollen has fairly high levels of thiamine, riboflavin, nicotinic acid, pyridoxine, pantothenic acid, biotin, folic acid and vitamin B_{12}. He has stated, 'It is apparent that pollens, as far as water-soluble vitamins are concerned, must be regarded as a product of exceptionally high nutritive value' (Lunden, 1954).

The B Vitamins

There are eight different B vitamins and they work best in conjunction with each other. All the B complex vitamins are water-soluble, so a daily intake is vital. In theory, these may be obtained from the average diet. However, as is becoming increasingly clear, modern farming methods, preservatives and many other factors rob our foods of their nutrients. It is therefore advisable to ensure optimum levels by taking either a B complex vitamin supplement or royal jelly, which has relatively high levels. Remember, the B vitamins work together so, unless individual B vitamins have been prescribed by a practitioner for specific conditions (see below), avoid taking numerous individual vitamins.

Thiamine (vitamin B1)

Thiamine is known as the 'morale vitamin' because of the beneficial effects it has on the nervous system and morale. People with heart disease have been found to have lower than normal levels of thiamine in their heart muscle.

Benefits
- Ensures mental alertness.
- Vital for the release of energy from carbohydrates, fats and alcohol.
- During pregnancy, thiamine ensures the correct growth of the foetus.
- Ensures good digestion.

Deficiency symptoms
- Severe deficiency is now extremely rare in the West.
- Minor deficiency will lead to mental problems, such as loss of concentration, depression, irritability and memory loss. Weight loss and tummy upsets also occur.
- Probably the earliest symptom is continuous nausea.

Who may need to supplement?
- The elderly.
- Pregnant women.
- Smokers.
- Alcoholics.
- People under physical or mental stress.
- People who have a high carbohydrate intake.
- Those convalescing from surgery or an accident.

Therapeutic uses
- Sciatica.
- Lumbago.
- Deters insect bites.

Riboflavin (vitamin B$_2$)

Riboflavin has a yellow colour and, as a result, has been used as a food colouring.

Benefits
- Riboflavin forms two essential coenzymes (flavin dinuleotide and flavin mononumleotide) that, together, are responsible for converting proteins, fats and sugars into substances the body can use.
- Important for healthy skin and hair.

Deficiency symptoms
- Cold sores.
- Burning, itchy eyes that tire easily and are sensitive to light.
- Dermatitis.
- Hair loss.

Who may need to supplement?
- Women on the Pill.
- Adults with irregular or poor eating habits.
- Vegetarians and vegans.

Therapeutic uses
- For sores and ulcers.
- For eye problems.
- For migraines (although there is no explanation for this).
- For muscle cramps.

Niacin (vitamin B₃)

Niacin comes in two forms: acid (nicotinic acid) and amide (nicotinamide) – neither of which has anything in common with nicotine. Niacin was also referred to as 'PP' because it prevented pellagra, a niacin-deficiency disease whose symptoms are diarrhoea, dermatitis and dementia.

Benefits
- The acid form – nicotinic acid – plays an important role in the nervous system and circulation.
- The amide form – nicotinamide – processes carbohydrates, fats and protein as part of the production of energy.

Deficiency symptoms
- Diarrhoea, dermatitis and dementia (pellagra).
- Nervous tension.

Who may need to supplement?
- Schizophrenics.
- Alcoholics.

Therapeutic uses
- Arthritis sufferers have found niacin supplementation can improve mobility.
- Alcoholics demonstrate the same type of mental disturbance as schizophrenics and both groups respond better to niacin supplementation in megadoses (strictly under medical supervision) than they do to many drug treatments.
- Taken under medical supervision, megadoses of niacin have been known to reduce blood cholesterol.

Pantothenic acid (vitamin B₅)

Its name comes from the Greek 'panthos', which means 'everywhere' and it is, indeed, widely found everywhere – in our body tissues and in plants.

Benefits
- Pantothenic acid is very important to the process of releasing energy from foods. This is because it is part of coenzyme A, which plays a major role in energy release.
- Pantothenic acid is used to make and renew our body tissues.
- It is vital for the production of antibodies (part of our immune system).

Deficiency symptoms
- 'Burning feet' syndrome.
- Tiredness.
- Depression.
- Loss of appetite.
- Cramps.
- Indigestion.
- Insomnia.

Who may need to supplement?
- Alcoholics.
- Women on the Pill.
- Pregnant women.
- Smokers.

Therapeutic uses
- To relieve nausea.
- To relieve PMS.

- To treat 'burning feet' syndrome.
- Skin disorders.

Pyridoxine (vitamin B6)

Pyridoxine is known as the 'women's vitamin' because it is particularly beneficial to women. Pyridoxine is essential to the production of adrenalin and insulin. High-protein diets increase the need for vitamin B6.

Benefits
- B6 is essential for energy production.
- B6 is vital for the nervous system.
- Involved in protein metabolism.

Deficiency symptoms
- Premenstrual syndrome.
- Seborrhoea (oily skin with crusts and scales) around the eyes, nose and mouth.
- Lowered white blood cell count.
- Swollen ankles, abdomen and fingers.

Who may need to supplement?
- Women on the Pill.
- Alcoholics.
- Breastfeeding women.
- Smokers.
- People with heart disease.
- Women following hormone replacement therapy.

Therapeutic uses
- Cystitis.
- Flu.
- Conjunctivitis.

Cobalamin (vitamin B12)

Vegans and vegetarians are likely to be short of vitamin B12 because it is available in meat products and does not normally occur in vegetables. Vitamin B12 was the last true vitamin to be classified. It is called cobalamin because it contains cobalt, an essential trace element.

Benefits
- Vitamin B12 maintains a healthy nervous system.
- Promotes growth in children.
- Needed for production of red blood cells.
- Maintains the protective 'myelin sheath' around the nerves.
- Used to metabolize fatty acids.

Deficiency symptoms
- Pernicious anaemia, which is a shortfall of red blood cells (if enough folic acid is taken, the symptoms of pernicious anaemia are hidden until irreversible neurological damage is done).
- Menstrual problems.
- Listlessness.
- Tremors.

Who may need to supplement?
- Vegans and vegetarians.
- Alcoholics.
- Pregnant women.
- The elderly.
- Smokers.
- People who take medicines for stomach ulcers and similar.

Therapeutic uses
- People with moodiness and paranoia respond positively to vitamin B_{12}.
- Relief from symptoms such as mental fatigue and memory impairment.
- Detoxifies chemicals in tobacco smoke.

Folic Acid

Folic acid was so named because it is found in green leaves, or foliage. Low folic acid intake during pregnancy is associated with spina bifida. Women intending to start a family are now advised to supplement with folic acid before becoming pregnant.

Benefits
- Folic acid is involved in passing on the genetic code to offspring.
- It is involved in the formation of healthy cells.
- It is needed for DNA production and cell division.

Deficiency symptoms
- Anaemia, the symptoms of which are weakness, insomnia, forgetfulness, mental confusion and breathlessness.

Who may need to supplement?
- Pregnant women, because the foetus makes large demands for folic acid.
- Coeliacs.
- The elderly, who tend to have poorer diets or impaired absorption.
- Alcoholics.

Therapeutic uses
- Schizophrenia is known to respond positively when folic acid is taken together with vitamin B_6.

Biotin

Biotin, a water-soluble member of the B complex of vitamins, is sometimes referred to as 'Vitamin H' or 'coenzyme R'. A substance in raw egg whites combines with biotin to make the toxic ingredients in egg whites ineffective.

Benefits
- Biotin is required to process carbohydrates, energy and fats.
- Biotin prevents premature greying and balding.

Deficiency symptoms
- Biotin deficiency is rare in humans, unless large amounts of raw eggs have been consumed.
- Scaly dermatitis in adults or 'cradle cap' in infants.
- Hair loss.
- More common in babies than adults.

Who may need to supplement?
- Infants suffering from dermatitis.
- Pregnant women.

Therapeutic uses
- To treat cradle cap.
- To alleviate dermatitis and eczema.
- Thought to relieve candida.

The only foods that contain more pantothenic acid than bee pollen are beef brain, hens' eggs, cauliflower, Irish potatoes and tomatoes. Bee pollen's nicotinic acid levels are higher than those of dried beans and peas and almost the same as beef and liver, its thiamine content being almost the same as beef liver. There is a similar level of riboflavin in bee pollen as in dried skimmed cow's milk, but no other plant source can match it, apart from certain yeasts.

Bee pollen is also comprised of bioflavonoids which give it its distinctive colour. There are a number of these, including quercetin, rutin, kaempferol, isohamnetin, naringenin, luteolin, apigenin, diosmetrin, myrectin and pollenin. Bioflavonoids are of particular benefit to us as they have been found to have an antioxidant effect, helping to scavenge free radicals, the 'rogue' and unstable oxygen molecules that can go on the rampage and destroy our body cells and tissues. Bioflavonoids are commonly found in foods high in vitamin C.

Vitamin C is another powerful antioxidant nutrient in its own right and it, too, is found in bee pollen. Like the B vitamins, it is water-soluble. Robert Delperee, in a paper he wrote in 1961, describes it thus: 'Stimulating antitoxic and antihaemorrhagic effects; beneficial against colds, respiratory distress; required for the efficient use and metabolism of calcium (promotes the effect of calcium, eliminates toxic phenomena arising as a consequence of absorbing too strong a dose of calcium); reduces hypercalcification induced by excessive doses of vitamin D'.

Other vitamins found in bee pollen include the carotenes, vitamins D and E and, when pollen is fermented (also known as bee bread), vitamin K.

The following enzymes have been identified:

- amylase
- diastase
- saccharase
- pectase
- phosphatase
- catalase
- disphorase
- cozymase
- cytochrome systems
- lactic dehydrogenase
- succinic dehydrogenase
- 24 oxidoreductases
- 21 transferases
- 33 hydrolases
- 11 lysases
- 5 isomerases
- pepsin
- trypsin.

Other bee pollen 'ingredients' include pectin, nucleic acids, waxes, resins, plant growth factors, xanthophylls, brassins, crocetin, zeaxanthin, pentosans and lecithin.

Small wonder that bee pollen has been described as a 'complete food'. In the words of Robert Delperee, 'It is possible to let several successive generations [of mice] be born and live without the least sign of distress while nourishing them exclusively on pollen. The optimum of vigour and resistance to poor health and disease was obtained by adding a mixture of 20 per cent bee pollen to their feed. Bee pollen is rich in rare and precious nutritive compounds; it works in a deep and lasting fashion ... The percentage of revivifying and rejuvenating elements in bee pollen is remarkable, far exceeding those present in brewer's yeast and wheat germ ... Bee pollen contains all the essential components of life ... ' (Delperee, 1961).

These sentiments were echoed in a lecture by Doctor Gunther Vorwhol at a German Apiarist Convention in Sontra, Germany, in the late 1980s. Entitled 'Pollen and Honey', his lecture proclaimed:

Bee pollen is known to be a very protein-rich food for man. Besides all the essential amino acids present in bee pollen, many scientific studies confirm that the vitamin balance can be improved by eating this complete food from the bee hive. And there are other interesting active substances present in bee pollen as well. It offers rutin, for instance, which favourably influences the permeability of capillaries. Not to mention the important hormonal factors, the substances which act like the oestrogenic or gonadatropic hormones which so greatly aid the human reproductive functions, both male and female. I should also point out the bacteria-inhibiting effects of the pollen collected by bees.

Science teaches that bee pollen contains numerous substances which make it a healthy protein-rich nutritious food. Additionally, there are numerous reports from medical experience which show the benefits of bee pollen exceeds that of a simple food item. Repeated reports have been published about the positive influence of the ingestion of bee pollen in the case of prostate difficulties, the favourable influence bee pollen causes in cases of infertility, both male and female, and how it erases menopausal complaints. Because of the proven activity of the hormones in bee pollen, these cases are quite plausible.

It is time to focus world attention on the utilization of bee pollen, the protein food of the bees. Bee pollen belongs with the protein-rich plant materials. Protein-rich pollen types are preferred by the bees. The protein content of blended bee pollen contains all the essential amino acids we must ingest every day, as the human body cannot produce them. The essential amino acids occur in pollen in free form, as well as bound to protein. Mixed bee pollens correspond favourably to other valuable protein foods, including eggs, cheese and soybeans. And the bees do most of the work. As beekeepers, we must harvest more and more of this food from the hive and teach others to do the same, especially in the malnourished and starving areas of the world. Bee pollen can be the answer to worldwide hunger.

And if this is not enough to convince you of the nutritional benefits of bee pollen, perhaps the following will dispel any lingering doubts:

Honeybee pollen is the richest source of vitamins found in nature in a single food. Even if bee pollen had none of its other vital ingredients, its content of rutin alone would justify taking at least a teaspoon daily, if for no other reason than strengthening the capillaries. Pollen is extremely rich in rutin and may have the highest content of any source, plus a very high content of the nucleics, RNA and DNA.

Taranov, 1977

Bee pollen is a complete food and contains many elements that products of animal origin do not possess. Bee pollen is more rich in proteins than any animal source. It contains more amino acids than beef, eggs, or cheese of equal weight. Bee pollen is particularly concentrated in all elements necessary for life.

Alain Callais, 1974

Bee pollen is the finest, most perfect food. It is a giant germ-killer in which bacteria simply cannot exist. The health-restoring properties of honeybee pollen have been proven time

and time again. Honeybee pollen not only builds up strength
and energy in the body, but gives increased resistance to infection.

Dr G. J. Binding, in Brown,
How to Live the Millennium: The bee pollen bible

3

Propolis – Better Than Antibiotics

Propolis

You will recall from Chapter 2 that this resinous compound is used by bees to seal their hives from outside threats and to sterilize the brood cells before the eggs are laid. It now seems that it has the potential to become a major medical discovery, as important as penicillin. Indeed, it is even being suggested that propolis has qualities that outrank penicillin, streptomycin and tetracycline in its effects. These three established antibiotics are derived from unsophisticated microorganisms whereas propolis is extracted by the bees from trees, which are much further along in evolutionary terms.

Dr K. Lund Aagaard of Denmark has described it as follows:

Propolis is one of the most efficient bee products from the viewpoint of active principles transmitted from plant to man. Its main sources are the substances collected from poplar or *Salicaceae* buds. The bees add salivary secretions and wax to the resinous raw substance. Nineteen substances of different chemical structure have been identified so far.

Aagaard, The Natural Product Propolis: The way to health

So, how does it work? It is thought to stimulate the immune system and to kill infectious organisms (bacteria, fungi and viruses) or to render them ineffective.

It stimulates the immune system by enhancing the actions of the phagocytes, which are the white blood cells that destroy invading germs. Experiments on mice exposed to infection have shown that, after having been injected with propolis, at least twice as many phagocytes were available to fight off the infection than in the mice not injected with propolis. In addition, propolis stimulates the thymus gland, which contains developing lymphocytes, other white blood cells involved in the immune system and which fight against infection and illness. Its action has been described as initiating the 'intracellular digestion of staphylococci (poison-forming substances) and promotes a cleansing of cells and bloodstream' (Balalykina, *Propolis: Its Antibacterial and Therapeutic Properties*).

That propolis acts in this way on staphylococci has been confirmed by recent research conducted in the laboratory of Polish researchers Scheller, Tustanowski and Paradowski. They determined that an alcohol-propolis solution proved effective in the treatment of dermatitis and gynaecological infections.

During their test, they compared the sensitivity of bacteria and attempted to show the possible correlation between their respective sensitivities to propolis and antibiotics. They tested 56 different strains of the bacteria staphylococcus. The antibiotics used were penicillin, ampicillin, meticillin, streptomycin, cloramphenicol, teramycin, erythrocyn, myacyn and sulphathiazole.

The study found that on almost all strains, the sensitivity to propolis was higher than to the antibiotics tested. Even strains with low sensitivity to propolis exhibited a wide range in degree of sensitivity to antibiotics and a general reduction of their sensitivity to antibiotics was recorded (Brown, *How to Live the Millennium: The bee pollen bible*).

If you find the above explanation rather technical, consider the following lesson from the hive. It has been noted that if a mouse enters a hive, it is first stung to death and, because it is too heavy to be removed by the bees, it is first covered in propolis and then shrouded with beeswax. This prevents decay and becomes a protection against micro-organisms. It is this example that may help us understand how a virus can be encased by propolis and rendered harmless in our bodies. What is more, unlike antibiotics, the micro-organisms cannot build tolerance against propolis.

Another way in which propolis benefits the immune system is to prevent viruses from entering the cells in our body and making us ill. In some way, propolis prevents the body's cells from being tricked by the invading virus into taking off the virus' outer layer and exposing the infecting contents within. It is when the virus manages to break through a cell's own protective layer that the infection takes hold. The cell is then forced to replicate the virus.

One explanation for propolis' ability to protect the immune system in this way that has been put forward is that propolis contains bioflavonoids. Bioflavonoids have an antioxidant capacity, which, as we saw earlier, means that they are able to counteract free radicals, those rampant and unstable oxygen molecules that can damage cells and body tissue. Bioflavonoids have also been credited with the ability to heal small blood vessels and to act as a vasodilator (a substance that causes dilation of the blood vessels). Other reports have described their effectiveness in treating such disorders as 'rheumatic fever, spontaneous abortions and miscarriages, high blood pressure, respiratory infections, haemorrhoids, cirrhosis of the liver, etc.'

Another study conducted in Sarajevo by Professor

Osmanagic, mentioned in *The Healing Power of Pollen with Propolis and Royal Jelly*, further tested the hypothesis that propolis helps to protect us from viruses. During a flu epidemic in the town, he gave a group of students and teachers at a nursing training college propolis, which they were to take diluted with honey every day for some 40 to 50 days. These people were symptom-free at the start of the study. Only about a tenth of the students taking propolis caught the flu virus, whereas a quarter of those who did not take propolis caught it. The ratio among the teachers was even more impressive – only 1 in 25 of those taking propolis was ill.

The fact that propolis also kills bacteria and fungal infections has been demonstrated in laboratory testing. In 1960, the Russian scientist Dr Rabinovic (the Russians have extensively researched these properties) collected some of the infective microbes from tuberculosis patients. Under carefully controlled conditions, these microbes were allowed to multiply. He then looked to see what effect propolis had on their further development. He found that propolis actually stopped the increase of the organisms. Other studies have found that the antibacterial characteristics of propolis are retained even after many years, assuming correct storage.

Dr Lindenfelser, in 1967, studied 39 types of bacteria, 39 types of fungi and 2 yeasts and evaluated how effective 15 samples of propolis were against them. He was able to report that propolis is highly effective against 25 of the 39 types of bacteria and 20 of the 39 species of fungi. Propolis did not have much effect on the yeasts. Some of the propolis samples worked better than others and this was accounted for by the observation that they had different bioflavonoid contents.

Dr Lavie, also from Russia, has identified seven antibiotics in bee products, including propolis, *The Healing Power of Pollen with Propolis and Royal Jelly*). Propolis is made up of 50 to 55 per cent resin and balsam, 30 per cent wax, 8 to 10 per cent oils and 5 per cent solid material. Propolis also contains the B complex vitamins and vitamins A, C, H and P (the bioflavonoids) as well as trace minerals.

K. Lund Aagaard, a well-known naturopath and medical writer from Denmark, published a paper that reviewed some of the extensive research conducted in Scandinavia on the properties of propolis. In it he states, 'During my long practice, I had the opportunity to examine certain afflictions and often experimented with propolis in its natural form. I obtained relevant results [based on] experiments [that] involved more than 50,000 persons all across Scandinavia' (Brown, *How to Live the Millennium: The bee pollen bible*).

He also cites its effectiveness in treating a wide range of conditions such as swelling of the large intestine, infection of the urinary tract, swelling of the throat, gout, open wounds , colds, influenza, bronchitis, gastritis, diseases of the ears, periodontal disease, intestinal infections, ulcers, eczema eruptions, pneumonia, arthritis, lung disease, stomach virus, headaches, Parkinson's disease, bile infections, sclerosis, warts, conjunctivitis and hoarseness.

Propolis is on the market in a number of forms – as raw chips (useful for sore throats and coughs), as toothpaste (to treat halitosis, gum disorders, toothaches and as a teeth whitener), in capsule form (for internal problems such as ulcers and digestive disorders), as lozenges (for mouth sores), in tinctures (for ear infections or cuts and tonsillitis) and in ointment (to treat burns, corns, eczema and psoriasis).

Old Time Remedies

Remedies from the past using propolis give us clues as to how we might apply propolis to ailments today.

Corns
Coat the affected area with a thick layer of propolis and cover (a plaster will do). Apply more propolis each night before retiring. In just a few days, the corn should soften and can soon be easily removed.

Sore throat
Put a lump of propolis in your mouth and let it dissolve. The infection usually clears up overnight.

Minor burns
Prepare an infusion of propolis by pouring boiling water over a lump of propolis. Let it brew. Pour the liquid into a jar and keep for whenever necessary. In the event of a burn, bathe the area immediately with the infusion.

    Source: R. Brown, *How to Live the Millennium: The bee pollen bible* (Hohm Press, 1994).

4

Royal Jelly

It is not surprising when you consider the effect that this food has on the size of the queen bee that royal jelly has been found to have a similar influence on other animals when fed experimentally with royal jelly. Fruit flies, pigs, cockerels and chickens became larger, had a longer lifespan and were more fertile. In fact, the laying capacity of the chickens was twice that of those chickens not fed royal jelly.

As for humans, there is well-respected scientific evidence that royal jelly can work for us, too, and right throughout life. Undernourished babies have been found to improve in just two weeks when fed royal jelly – they gain weight and their overall health improves. These results have been repeated in older children, too, and in adults. The nervous conditions of mental patients have been stabilized. Ulcer patients have also benefited, as have those suffering from Parkinson's disease and Bueger's disease, arthritis, leukaemia and arteriosclerosis. Royal jelly has seen many women successfully through the menopause, with some even being able to conceive again. Its rejuvenating properties have helped many elderly people, too.

The composition of royal jelly is almost identical to that of bee pollen as it is from bee pollen that royal jelly is made. However, its carbohydrate content is greater, although the three main sugars are the same – fructose, glucose and sucrose. As for the B complex vitamins, the level of pantothenic acid in royal jelly is 17 times higher than that of bee pollen. It is rich in natural hormones and has a high concentration of proteins, including cysteine, lysine and arginine. Another component is acetylcholine, which is important for transmitting nerve messages throughout the body and is involved in the production of glandular secretions. Royal jelly also contains 10-hydroxy–2-decanoic acid, which is not found in bee pollen. This acid is manufactured from pollen and nectar sucrose by the nurse bees for feeding to the larvae. It acts as an antibiotic, fighting bacteria and fungal infections.

Royal jelly has generous quantities of bee pollen and the process of persorption has been found to apply here, too. It also contains all of the 30 amino acids known in nature, including the 8 'essential amino acids, which cannot be manufactured by the body – they must be obtained through the diet. The B complex and C vitamins are present in plentiful supply and trace minerals are there, too. About 3 per cent of its contents has confounded analysis, which means that it cannot be replicated, but also that no vitamin/mineral supplement can act on the body in exactly the same way as royal jelly.

The following excerpts are taken from a paper by Dr A. Saenz, formerly Head of the Laboratory of the Anti-Rabies Institute of Montevideo, Uruguay, and subsequently a member of the staff at the Pasteur Institute in Paris. This paper provides an excellent overview of the benefits and effects of royal jelly and covers the work of other scientists.

He says, 'Each day man enlarges the therapeutic arsenal which he uses to battle against senescence [ageing], the term of his lifecycle [longevity], and against diseases which disturb his biological equilibrium for as long as he exists.

The use of royal jelly has spread widely and continues to be of interest more and more to the scientist, the biologist and the physician. (Saenz, 1984). Indeed, during the last ten years, a number of studies have demonstrated the existence of important nutrients, the presence of which could partly explain the remarkable and mysterious properties of royal jelly. Among the prime ones are the water-soluble B vitamins identified by Dr Saenz in his paper – thiamine (B_1), riboflavin (B_2), niacin(B_3), pyridoxine (B_6), biotin, inositol and pantothenic acid (B_5) (see pages 15–23).

Commenting on the therapeutic effects of royal jelly, he states that 'as a biogenetic product [it], has been in use since 1952 in human clinical practice. Its field of action is becoming progressively extended, thanks to the research of that great French biologist, Boyer de Belvefer. Royal jelly has rendered valuable aid to a great number of sick people ... '. The paper also focuses on the fact that, in general, in all states of convalescence, royal jelly benefits the body and that stress, physical or mental exhaustion, so frequent in modern life, are rapidly corrected by treatment with royal jelly.

Arteriosclerosis

With regard to arteriosclerosis, he observes that 'the action of royal jelly in arteriosclerosis is extremely interesting and rests on experimental verification'. Quoting other researchers such as Russ, Eder and Ban, he emphasizes the relationship arteriosclerosis has with high levels of cholesterol. Arteriosclerosis is the consequence of a disturbed fat metabolism and worsens considerably with age. He concludes that, 'When those who are suffering from arteriosclerosis are subjected to royal jelly, it re-establishes normal activities of the metabolic process where lipoproteins originate'.

Varicose Veins

Dr Saenz goes on to suggest that royal jelly can have excellent results when used to treat varicose veins as well as lead to quite significant improvements in other disorders of the arteries.

Paediatrics

At the meeting of the Congress of Medicine at Bologna, Italy, leading experts Professor Malassi and Dr Grandi concluded that royal jelly ought to be part of the biological therapy for the feeding of premature infants. Various clinical trials have established the effectiveness of royal jelly as a general tonic, thus rapidly promoting necessary weight gain.

Neurology

In some cases, a satisfactory remission in Parkinson's disease has been obtained by sufferers taking royal jelly, including a marked reduction of the trembling caused by this disease, and experts now suggest that further studies should be carried out in order to understand the benefits royal jelly offers victims of neurological disorders.

Dermatology

Royal jelly acts as a bactericide and antibiotic while revitalizing the skin. Several specialists have employed royal jelly treatment with success in eczema, neurodermatitis and impetigo. Its use is most effective for skin ailments with a very alkaline pH. Royal jelly has an acidic pH and this re-establishes the acid mantle of the skin.

While we must acknowledge that we do not know enough

about the exact therapeutic properties of royal jelly, we need
to seriously look at the exciting potential of this wondrous
substance. Dr Saenz makes a pertinent observation: 'What is
astonishing from the biological viewpoint is royal jelly's
extreme concentration as compared to human blood plas-
ma. The beneficial action of royal jelly is due to the presence
of and the synergy between various substances harmonious-
ly bound to one another and mutually reinforcing their
effect'. In other words, royal jelly could enable a biological
balance to be established, helping us mitigate the ageing
process itself.

5

Who May Benefit?

As indicated in earlier chapters, bee products are of benefit for a wide range of needs and across the whole age range, from the very young to the elderly. However, there are particular groups of people for whom bee products are a source of extra help. They are the very young, women, those who are ill, athletes and the elderly.

Children

Of particular benefit to children is royal jelly. You will recall from the last chapter that undernourished babies who were given this food gained weight as well as experiencing an overall improvement in their health.

One study that demonstrated this was undertaken in Florence by the Department of Clinical Paediatrics at the University there. Altogether, 42 children ranging from premature babies to undernourished children, as well as children suffering from spasms, were given royal jelly. They were reported to have responded favourably to the treatment. Almost all had an increase in appetite and they looked visibly better after just 20 days. Blood tests revealed that their red blood count was up, and for those children who suffered from low white blood cell counts, it was found that their counts had returned to normal. Also, proteins were better absorbed from their food into the bloodstream after treatment, *The Healing Power of Pollen with Propolis and Royal Jelly*, and see for details of other research covered in this and the following chapter).

An animal study on rats conducted in 1977 by scientists from the Egyptian National Research Centre monitored the growth of baby female rats given royal jelly against the growth of those fed normally. The average weight of the rats to begin with was 37 g (approximately 1¼ oz). Four weeks later, the rats that had been fed royal jelly were found to have increased in weight to 79 g (about 3 oz). Those fed normally weighed only 60 g (2¼ oz) after the same period. Sexual maturity also took place earlier in the group fed royal jelly .

There is anecdotal evidence that royal jelly has a calming influence and may therefore be of benefit for those children (and their parents!) who are hyperactive. This applies equally to children who suffer from eczema.

Bee pollen may also be of benefit to children and, indeed, royal jelly contains bee pollen. Children are exposed to many sources of infection at school and at play and there is a good argument for taking it as a preventive measure, particularly in preparation for winter. It has been suggested that a two- to three-month course of bee pollen in the autumn months will ward off many of winter's ills.

If your child succumbs to a sore throat or a cold, then taking a combination of vitamin C and propolis in the form of lozenges or as a tincture for gargling and swallowing may help to reduce the unpleasant symptoms and may even cure the illness. In fact, propolis salve has been used since 1962 at the St Petersburg's K. A. Rachfuss Children's Hospital on children with infected wounds or on newborns with tissue disorders with some success.

Women

Bee products are valuable to women at all the major stages of their lives – through menstruation, pregnancy and childbirth, the menopause and into old age.

Many women suffer from period problems or premenstrual syndrome. Evening primrose oil, once scoffed at by the medical establishment, has now become one of the standard treatments for this disorder. Royal jelly, too, has a part to play in helping to alleviate the condition, particularly as it is rich in the B vitamins that are especially important for regulating the menstrual cycle. It can also help to counteract the acne many women are prone to at certain times in the cycle as these same vitamins, together with vitamin C and amino acids, are beneficial to the health of the skin.

Period pains themselves may be reduced by taking royal jelly and there is some scientific evidence to corroborate these claims. In Eastern Europe, a trial was conducted involving two groups of 30 girls aged between 18 and 22 years. The characteristics of the first group were that they were underweight and had irregular and very painful periods. There were no menstrual problems among those in the second group, apart from painful periods. The groups were further divided so that half of the girls in each group received a placebo (a pill containing non active ingredients) and the other half one capsule daily of Melbrosia PLD (a royal jelly and bee pollen compound). After two months, three-quarters of the underweight girls gained between 1.25 and 2.75 kg (2 and 6½ lbs) whereas only a quarter those in the second group did so. As for the menstrual pains, out of all the girls taking Melbrosia, only two failed to show any improvement. In the group taking the placebo, only six reported an improvement (Pokrajcic and Osmanagic, 1976).

Once a woman becomes pregnant, there may be other

discomforts that affect her. They may be all or any of the following – cramps, sleeplessness, depression, fatigue and, of
course, the infamous morning sickness. Royal jelly has been
said to help to relieve some or all of these miseries without
the worries accompanying the taking of potentially harmful
drugs. There is little scientific research to back up these
claims, although there is plenty of anecdotal evidence. Royal
jelly also has the advantage of restoring nutrients lost
through excessive vomiting, should it occur. Many women
who have had morning sickness have found that they
stopped experiencing such nausea after they started taking
royal jelly.

Unfortunately, women's gynaecological problems do not
end after childbirth. The next major phase in a woman's life
is the menopause, also called 'the change'. Some women sail
through it, but many others experience pronounced symptoms that can cause anxiety and embarrassment. Bee pollen
and royal jelly together have been found to be especially useful in relieving these symptoms.

Dr Bogdan Tekavcic of the Ljubljiana Centre for Gynaecology has focused his attention on the problems of older
women. He took a group of 74 women, aged between 40 and
55, who were beginning to show signs of the menopause,
although they were still having periods. Half of them took
the bee pollen and royal jelly supplement on an empty stomach for two months and the rest were given a placebo. In the
first group, 20 of the women unexpectedly lost weight, while
only 7 gained weight. Only four lost weight in the group
taking the placebo. As for the rest of the menopausal symptoms, their severity was measured by a Climacteric Index
and it was found that 35 out of the 38 taking the supplement
felt a substantial improvement in their symptoms. In fact, in
14 of the cases, their indices fell below 10, which meant that
they were virtually symptom free.

Dr Tekavcic was able to repeat these results in a study of older women, aged from 40 to 65, who had not menstruated for at least a year but were still experiencing unpleasant symptoms. These studies were subsequently confirmed by Professor Osmanagic of the Gynaecological Department at Sarajevo University, whose own trial covered a period of six months. He wanted to see especially whether such symptoms as hot flushes, perspiration, headaches and palpitations could be relieved. He found that 45 per cent of the women were able to record 'very good' results, while another 45 per cent evaluated the results as 'good'. The rest (only four women) had only 'slight' improvement (Osmanagic, 1972).

There are many other afflictions women can face – erosion and irritation of the cervix, cellular disorders and vaginal disorders. Propolis has been used successfully as a salve in such instances. Experts at the Clinic for Obstetrics and Gynaecology at the Crimea Medical Institute found that when propolis was applied directly to the eroded surface of the cervix, after only four days the erosion had begun to heal. There was almost complete healing after 12 days, propolis having been applied daily. In almost 98 per cent of the women treated, there was some healing.

Members of the Department of Obstetrics and Gynaecology in Goczalkowice Zdroj in Poland reported that propolis vaginal tablets were used to heal inflammations of the neck of the womb and vagina. Propolis was also found by Drs Osmanagic, Mujezinovic and Pokrajcic to be helpful in relieving the symptoms of dysmenorrhoea (painful or difficult periods). Itching, dryness and discomfort from haemorrhoids have all been found to heal in a short time when bee propolis salve is applied.

Apart from gynaecological problems, many women suffer from the occasional bout of cystitis (although men can also be affected, this is less common). Some women, however, have repeated attacks and are at their wits end in knowing how to treat it as the antibiotics usually prescribed can be ineffective. Royal jelly, with its own antibiotic properties and containing the vitamins and minerals that help to counter-act the infection, has been found by some to be the cure they have been seeking for this painful complaint, which some-times has plagued them for several years.

Athletes

When one thinks of the thousands of trips and the miles cov-ered by the bee in searching for just the right nectar or pollen, one begins to wonder how such a small creature finds the stamina to carry out such tasks. The answer must, of course, lie in the food it eats – honey and pollen. No wonder, then, that when athletes have searched for a drug-free boost to their athletic performance, they have turned to bee prod-ucts and bee pollen in particular.

Honey was used by the athletes of Ancient Greece to pro-vide energy immediately before a competition. In 1951, the Sports College in Canada began to look seriously at whether or not honey had a part to play in providing much-needed energy for their athletes, without side-effects. They set up a series of tests and collated information from other sources and honey was found to come top. Lloyd Perivale, writing about this research in *American Bee Journal* in 1955 stated that, 'Athletes participating in endurance tests showed better performance levels when fed two tablespoonfuls of honey 30 minutes before the test began'.

Since the 1970s, bee pollen has been the focus of atten-tion. In 1967, Finland could only boast one runner in the 100 top world runners. In the 1972 Olympics, however, the Finnish ratings had increased dramatically to 39. They

attributed the improvement in performance to taking bee
pollen as part of their training programme, as much as six
to ten tablets daily during training and four to six before a
competition. The reason given for such high doses was that
runners of that calibre need to take in about 5,000 calories
a day – difficult to achieve in a country where the climate
does not allow for the consumption of sufficient fresh food
all year round. There would also be insufficient time for the
digestion of the sorts of meals required to provide such a
high calorie intake. Lord Millar, a British nutritionist,
looked at the blood of a group of Finnish runners and found
that their average red blood count had increased from
11–13 grams per 100 millilitres to 15.5–17 grams per
100 millilitres in 1972, although he could not say categor-
ically that the increase was due to the bee pollen intake
(Lyngheim and Scagnetti, *Bee Pollen: Nature's miracle health
food*).

Also in the early 1970s, a symposium held in Sweden to
evaluate the effect of bee pollen on athletes heard how bee
pollen helped nine major Italian football teams (amateur,
semi-professional and professional) improve their perfor-
mances. The doctors attached to the teams concluded, after
measuring the changes in their breathing and physical resistance, that in almost all cases, the players' general state of
health had improved and they were less susceptible to
fatigue. Indeed, football trainers found that bee pollen helped
players to increase their weight – an important benefit as
footballers have a tendency to lose weight (Lyngheim and
Scagnetti, *Bee Pollen: Nature's miracle health food*).

Once the news spread about the success of the Finnish
athletes, other countries sought to try out bee pollen for
themselves. British athletes followed suit and were reporting
that bee pollen helped them to reach the peak of condition
for the Montreal Olympics and many American track

runners claimed that bee pollen was instrumental in helping them and their teams to win championship races. Mohammed Ali himself maintained that a vitamin and mineral cocktail containing honey and bee pollen is what enabled him to outfight Leon Spinks, a much younger man, in 1978. Trainers have claimed a significant reduction in the number of colds suffered by athletes, which has meant fewer lost training days and better performance.

It needs to be acknowledged that, despite these cheering examples, there have been studies that have failed to support these conclusions and it is clear that more research is needed. However, let us not leave out of the picture the antibiotic benefits of propolis for the sportsman or woman. In 1984, in Sarajevo, the Institute for Sports Medicine treated 112 injuries using propolis salve. These injuries were sustained through participation in a number of sports. The age range of those treated was between 17 and 25 years and 77 per cent were males, 23 per cent females. They were seen and treated either the same day as the injury or the following day and further applications of propolis salve were administered during the next two to five days. After just one hour, those treated found that their pain was relieved. Inflammation went down on the second day and, after three days, most of them said that they no longer suffered from pain. They were able to resume their activities after five to seven days.

The Elderly

It is in this group that significant results have been achieved by means of supplementation with bee products. Older people are often poorly nourished for two reasons. First, the body loses some of its ability to absorb nutrients from the diet as it ages and, second, the elderly often consume foods that have been nutritionally depleted through processing.

They are just the people who need a readily absorbed source of extra vitamins and minerals.

Bee pollen and royal jelly have been found to be the two most helpful bee products for this age group. A French study was conducted by Dr Jacques DuBrisay, who was at the time a consultant to the Ministry of Social Affairs. The study looked into the efficacy of the product Cernelle, containing 6 mg of fat-soluble and 120 mg of water-soluble bee pollen extract. A total of 48 males took part whose symptoms involved severe loss of appetite together with no real desire to eat, mental and physical exhaustion and the loss of the will to live. They were divided randomly into two groups. The average age of group A was 70 and of group B 72. No one knew who was receiving the bee pollen product or the placebo. They were given four capsules daily for four weeks.

The results of the trial were graded from 'very good' through 'good', 'fair' and 'poor' to 'nil'. For those who received the bee pollen capsules, the gradings were:

- 54.17 per cent (13) 'very good'
- 41.66 per cent (10) 'good'
- 4.17 per cent (1) 'fair'.

As for group B, the group receiving the placebo, the results were:

- 12.5 per cent (3) 'fair'
- 45.84 per cent (11) 'poor'
- 41.66 per cent (10) 'nil'.

The bee pollen cured the symptoms of general weariness, apathy, a desire for death, listlessness, no interest in getting out of bed or getting dressed, no desire to read and, indeed, wanting nothing to do with their surroundings.

As for their feelings of fatigue, 83.3 per cent of group A found that their fatigue lifted and 75 per cent of them also found their appetite returning. No such reports were made by any of the men in group B. Weight gain also occurred in group A, but not in group B. Energy, strength, concentration and speed of performance were also enhanced in group A, but not in group B.

As for royal jelly, again there are anecdotal reports from elderly people who have experienced an improvement in their symptoms. Another French study, this time way back in 1957, by a Dr Betourne who injected royal jelly found that the results, according to his colleague Dr Chauvin, 'tend to prove that royal jelly has most salutary results in cases of debility and senility. Improvement becomes noticeable after only a few injections [and] seems lasting' (Chauvin, 1957).

It has been observed by those who take royal jelly regularly that they retain their youthful looks and it has been claimed that royal jelly actually slows down the ageing process. One of the reasons for this may be because it contains an amino acid called gamma globulin. This component of protein helps the body to attack bacteria, viruses and toxins, the combined effects of which contribute to the ageing process. Another amino acid in royal jelly, a gelatinous substance, has been identified as a forerunner of collagen, which is the body's 'cement', holding our cells together.

The Ill

A wide range of illnesses have been found to respond to bee products. Anaemia, for example, has been alleviated by taking royal jelly. Being rich in B vitamins, iron and manganese, royal jelly is said to 'improve the condition of the blood', which means that it is better able to carry oxygen and other nutrients around the body. In fact, in circumstances that give rise to debility, royal jelly, with its wide range of nutrients, is a good all-round tonic, helping those taking it get back on their feet.

Propolis, too, has been described as enhancing 'life energy'. John Diamond, former President of the International Academy of Preventive Medicine, stated in 1978 in *BK– Behavioural Kinesiology*:

> Of all the natural supplements I have tested, the one that seems to be the most strengthening to the thymus and hence the Life Energy, is bee resin, or bee propolis, a resin secreted by trees and then metabolized by the bees which bring it back to the hive to line the interior. This substance is the subject of considerable clinical research in several European countries. For many years it has proved to be effective against bacteria, viruses and fungi. We now know that the reason for this is that it activates the thymus gland and therefore the immune system.

As you will recall, it is the white blood cells that the thymus contains that protect us against illness and infection.

The addition of royal jelly to propolis has been found to enhance the antiviral effects of propolis. Researchers, B. Filipic and M. Likvar of the University of Sarajevo reported that, although high concentrations of royal jelly and propolis on their own have antiviral properties, 'a proper combination of royal jelly, propolis and honey had a very obvious antiviral effect, especially against influenza, even diluted 1:10.

The bioflavonoids in propolis have an effect rather like that of aspirin in that they can reduce the symptoms of pain and fever by blocking or inhibiting the enzymes that produce the chemicals in the body that give rise to those symptoms. The same bioflavonoids stimulate the production by the white blood cells of interferon, which itself combats disease and increases resistance to infection.

As for bee pollen, as we have seen, there is evidence that it is itself able to remedy a large number of health problems – loss of appetite, blood clotting, anaemia, weight loss, weakness, heart disease and respiratory infections. In the 1950s, Drs Chauvin and Lenormand found that bee pollen could improve overall health and, specifically regarding those who are ill or recovering from illness or operations, they stated that it was an 'ideal food' as it restores weight and energy. You will recall, too, that rutin, which is contained in bee pollen, is believed to strengthen the capillaries and help regulate the heartbeat as well as reducing bleeding time. The B vitamins present in bee pollen are beneficial in preventing and treating atherosclerosis.

An Austrian doctor, Dr Rudolf Frey of the Kornenburg Hospital, advocates the use of bee pollen for treating patients with psychological disorders, such as nervous conditions, sleeplessness, headaches, anxiety and loss of concentration. He observed that such patients were able to relax and therefore able to sleep better.

Recovery from illness or surgery can be particularly stressful and, at such times our resistance is low. Stress, particularly if it is prolonged, can actually deplete the body of nutrients and so increase the body's need for those nutrients. The pituitary and adrenal glands work overtime in an effort to counteract the effects of stress. These glands need pantothenic acid and the other B complex vitamins to be able to function and, as you now know, bee pollen contains all of these.

Bee products have been found to be effective in the treatment of gastrointestinal disorders, such as nausea, heartburn, hyperacidity and hypoacidity, abscesses or ulcers. Soviet scientists have observed that propolis, for example, helps to promote resistance to the formation of ulcers and speed up healing where there is already an ulcer. Bee pollen actually helps to improve cases of chronic diarrhoea and assists digestion, which, again, is especially important for those who are recovering from illness, as bee pollen has already gone through a process of digestion and its constituents are therefore able to be absorbed into the bloodstream much better.

There are conditions for which bee products have been found to be of particular benefit, either through prevention or even cure. These are described in the next chapter.

6

Bee Medicines for Prevention and Cure

Most bee products overlap in usefulness when it comes to treating particular ailments. This is because each one contains elements of the others. For example, royal jelly and natural, unprocessed honey contain bee pollen and propolis, royal jelly and bee pollen contain high levels of the B complex of vitamins. So, it is no coincidence that these products can assist in the treatment and cure of a number of different disorders and diseases.

Arthritis

You may be aware that there is more than one type of arthritis and that it is an umbrella term to describe a variety of conditions. The two forms that are most well known are osteoarthritis and rheumatoid arthritis. *Rheumatoid* arthritis usually starts as an inflammation of the synovial membrane, which covers the bones in the joints, helping them slide easily and may result in deposits in the joints and even deformity. *Osteoarthritis*, on the other hand, finds its source in the wear and tear of the joints during a person's lifetime.

One bee product that has been useful in relieving the symptoms of arthritis is also the most unlikely – bee venom.

Generally regarded as the stuff of old wives' tales, there is some scientific evidence that it works, although the results have been hard to replicate.

In the nineteenth century, an Austrian physician, Dr Philip Terc, used bee venom over a period of 40 years to treat hundreds of arthritis sufferers with a cure rate of 80 per cent. His interest in the healing properties of bee venom arose when he was cured of rheumatism after having been stung himself. Although initially considered as a crank, some other doctors did eventually try using it themselves in the treatment of arthritic patients with good results.

The Hungarian Dr Bodog F. Beck wrote in the 1930s about the use of bee venom for arthritis and rheumatism in his book *Bee Venom Therapy*. He died in the United States in 1942, but not before he managed to convince other US physicians to try it out. Subsequently, interest dwindled, although there were a few who kept the interest alive. There was a resurgence in 1962 when Dr Joseph Broadman wrote *Bee Venom: The natural curative for arthritis and rheumatism*. In it he claimed that he had successfully treated 40 cases of arthritis with bee venom.

Meanwhile, in Germany, England and Russia, bee venom was being analysed and was found to contain mellitin and apamin. It was also found that one of the enzymes present in the venom was able to highlight rheumatoid molecules present in the fluid that lubricates the joints. Bee venom acts on the pituitary and adrenal glands to increase their output of the body's own supply of cortisone, which is the body's own anti-inflammatory.

Whether bee venom actually cures arthritis or merely alleviates the symptoms is a matter of debate. Dr Joseph Saine of Montreal, Canada, stated:

With bee venom we did not only cure or relieve certain simple cases of rheumatism but also very chronic osteoarthritis and deformities and even fibrous ankylosis ... .Because of its properties of stimulation on antehypophysis and the suprarenal glands, bee venom enhances the body's defence, but unlike cortisone, without dangerous side-effects.

Lyngheim and Scagnetti,
Bee Pollen: Nature's miracle health food

However, Dr Gerald Weissman, an authority on arthritis who has conducted his own investigations into bee venom with rats artificially injected with a form of arthritis, concluded that venom does indeed stimulate the body's cortisone production, but that the most likely effect was that the symptoms of arthritis would be suppressed rather than cured.

Many people are afraid of bee stings and some are allergic to the venom, so they would be aghast if you suggested bee sting therapy as a cure or treatment for their ailments. Honey is likely be the more acceptable option. Reasons for its maybe being as effective as the venom itself are that honey has been found to contain the same neutralizing acids as are found in bee venom. Bees also use their stings in the process of preserving honey, so honey will contain bee venom anyway. If you are going to treat yourself with honey, you should ensure that you use only raw, uncooked, untreated and unpasteurized varieties. This is because processed honey has had the bee pollen removed and heating has killed the enzymes necessary to make it effective for treatment.

Surprisingly, beeswax has been found to have curative properties, and if you have arthritis, rubbing it on your hands and feet can be beneficial (healthfood shops stock the kind of beeswax that will help). This leads us to ask whether propolis has a part to play in the treatment of this disease as it, too, has an anti-inflammatory effect. A study in Austria conducted by Drs Eckl and Dworak supported its use for arthritis. This trial involved 56 people, 27 of whom suffered from arthritis, 18 from lumbago or other back pain, 8 from muscular pain and 3 from painful elbows. The patients were divided into two groups. One group received the propolis salve and the other a placebo ointment. After a few days, half of the group given propolis recorded 'impressive improvement' whereas only four of those given the placebo could say the same, and there were no side-effects.

Royal jelly, too, has been of help to sufferers. In the 1960s, Dr Barton-Wright conducted a study that demonstrated that rheumatoid and osteoarthritic patients benefited from an increase in pantothenic acid, which increased the mobility of their joints. Royal jelly contains pantothenic acid as well as pyridoxine, both of which are necessary for the repair and maintenance of the cartilage between the joints.

A case has been made for using bee pollen in the treatment of arthritis, too. Although there is little scientific evidence, there are many satisfied customers, as the producers can testify from their mailbags. Bee pollen has received praise for alleviating pain, maintaining mobility and decreasing the dependence on the drugs usually prescribed to ease this condition.

The Common Cold

One of the most well known home treatments for a cold is a combination of lemon and honey. The latter is said to soothe a sore throat, but can bee products actually prevent or cure a cold? One study that took place in 1967 in Sweden during an epidemic of flu answered this question in the affirmative. A heavy industrial company was concerned to minimize the number of days taken off by employees. It decided to give its employees tablets that contained 110 mg of bee pollen and 100 mg of aspirin. By the end of the epidemic, which lasted some 4 months, 510 employees had received a total of 908 packets of the product. Out of this large number of employees, only 9 came down with the flu.

You will recall from the previous chapter how trainers of athletes praised bee pollen for the reduction in training days lost due to colds and the paper presented by Drs Filipic and Likar of Yugoslavia which asserted that a combination of royal jelly and propolis inhibited the increase of the influenza virus. For royal jelly to be effective, however, it has to be natural and fresh.

An empirical study undertaken by Dr John Glomme of Oslo University, looking at the results of several studies into the effectiveness of bee pollen over a six-year period concluded that there was an overall reduction in the number of days being taken off sick and in visits to the doctor. The symptoms were also seen to be less severe and to last for less time.

Propolis works to relieve the symptoms of a cold or the flu by reducing the inflammation and infection in mucous membranes by means of the bioflavonoids it contains. These block the production of the prostaglandins responsible for these uncomfortable symptoms. As bioflavonoids also have an aspirin-like effect, this can help to prevent the other symptoms of pain and fever.

Again, many people who take royal jelly have reported that they have succumbed to colds far less than before and, when they do, their symptoms have been much less severe.

Frequent Infections

If you are one of those people who seems to catch everything that is going round, it could be that your immune system is functioning below par. Bee products are particularly valuable as a tonic, boosting the immune system. Propolis, for example, has been recognized as enhancing the ability of the white blood cells to scavenge for and engulf invading micro-organisms. The quantity of a protective protein in the blood, properdine, also increases and the cleansing powers of antibodies are enhanced. Interferon production is also increased by propolis and the thymus gland is activated, thereby strengthening immunity still further.

Bee pollen helps to reduce anaemia by helping to increase the production of red blood cells, as does royal jelly. The B complex of vitamins that they both contain are of importance in countering stress, which puts a strain on the immune system, thereby contributing to lowered resistance to infection. It seems, too, that royal jelly actually helps the heart, brain and liver tissue to use more oxygen from the blood, and this again contributes to better overall health.

Hair and Skin Problems

We all want to look our best and it can undermine our confidence when we find skin blemishes, our skin is irritated and when our hair seems to have lost its vitality. Honey and beeswax have long been ingredients in skin preparations as they are known to have cleansing and moisturizing properties. Royal jelly and bee pollen have also now found their way into the lists of ingredients of many natural cosmetics. This is because these bee products contain vitamins and minerals, hormones and amino acids, all of which help to 'feed' the skin.

Says Dr Lars-Erik Essen, a dermatologist from Halsinborg, Sweden, who has treated many of his patients for acne using bee pollen:

Through transcutaneous nutrition, bee pollen exerts a profound biological effect. It seems to prevent premature ageing of the cells and stimulates growth of new skin tissue. It offers effective protection against dehydration and injects new life into dry cells. It smooths away wrinkles and stimulates a life-giving blood supply to all skin cells.

The skin becomes younger looking, less vulnerable to wrinkles, smoother and healthier with the use of honeybee pollen. Taken internally or used externally, bee pollen exercises a suppressive effect on facial acne and is an important skin rejuvenator because it contains a high concentration of the nucleic acids, RNA and DNA, and a natural antibiotic.

Brown, How to Live the Millennium: The bee pollen bible

The B vitamins are of particular importance to maintaining clear, healthy skin and bee products are rich in these. Vitamin B_1 converts carbohydrates into energy. Lack of it can cause poor digestion and constipation, as well as headaches, a poor complexion, loss of appetite and heart trouble. A deficiency of B_2 (riboflavin) can result in cracked and rough skin. If there is insufficient B_3 (niacin), dermatitis may develop. Vitamin B_5 (pantothenic acid) helps the body to metabolize carbohydrates, fats and proteins. A diet rich in this vitamin helps you slow down the ageing process, retaining a more youthful appearance. Vitamin B_6 (pyridoxine) is needed for the growth, repair and replacement of body tissues, while B_7 (inositol) is essential for a healthy head of hair, as is B_8 (biotin). Vitamin B_9 (folic acid) and B_{12} (cobalamin) keep the blood supply healthy.

Another reason honey, bee pollen and royal jelly work is that they all retain moisture, which, in a moisturizer, will help to keep the skin free from wrinkles.

As mentioned above, for people suffering from acne, bee pollen is particularly useful as it has antiseptic and antibacterial properties and, if used in a lotion, this will meant that it will draw the impurities to the surface and promote rapid healing.

It has been suggested that bee pollen can restore hair growth because it is rich in cysteine, an amino acid that is an important component of hair. Whether it can actually cure baldness, however, is not so certain.

Propolis, too, is helpful for people suffering from other skin disorders, especially those that manifest themselves on the face, neck, thighs and so on. Drs T. V. Vinogradova and G. P. Zajceva have stated that propolis worked particularly well with patients who had recurrent skin disorders (Vinogradova and Zajceva, 1979).

One folk remedy for skin blemishes, using propolis, is as follows. 'Soak propolis onto a small pad of cotton wool. Smear all over facial spots such as acne, pimples, etc. Repeat as often as possible, especially after washing. Also good if left on overnight. Helps clear up blemishes within a short time' (Wade, *Propolis: Nature's energizer*).

An Austrian doctor, Dr Edith Lauda, has successfully treated patients suffering from persistent acne using propolis tincture and ointment. She relates the story of one woman who had suffered acne on her chin for 30 years. All other treatments had proved ineffective. Just two applications of propolis, however, left her skin trouble free, with some minor scarring (Wade, *Propolis: Nature's energizer*).

Carlson Wade lists some other 'tried and true' natural cosmetic remedies using bee pollen in his book *Bee Pollen and Your Health*. To deep cleanse your skin, mix 1 tablespoon of bee pollen grains with an egg yolk, half a cup of milk and half a ripe avocado. Apply with cotton wool balls.

To make a facial scrub, combine 1 tablespoon of bee pollen grains, half a mashed ripe avocado and half a cup of fine cornmeal. Having already thoroughly cleansed your face, rub this mixture onto troublesome areas, wipe off with a damp flannel and rinse with cold water to close the pores.

To exfoliate the skin of your body (but not your face), use a mixture of 2 tablespoons of bee pollen grains, half a ripe avocado, mashed, and half a cup of table salt. Rub this all over your body, and then shower it off.

If your skin is in need of a pick-me-up, try this rejuvenating cream. Make it and use it straight away as it does not keep very well. Mix 2 teaspoons of bee pollen grains, a quarter of a ripe avocado, mashed, and 2 tablespoons instant dried skimmed milk mixed with 2 tablespoons of water in a blender until you have a pale green cream. Apply the cream to your cleansed face and leave it on until your skin begins to tighten. Add another layer. When it is dry (about ten minutes later), wash it off with lukewarm water and a flannel and then rinse well.

For a longer-lasting lotion that you can keep in your refrigerator for whenever you need an astringent for a quick facial or to liven up a dull and tired complexion, you should combine the following. For every cup of strained, fresh lemon juice, add 1 teaspoon of bee pollen grains and half a cup of water. Shake it well.

For an all-purpose moisturizer, mash a very ripe banana with half an avocado and 2 teaspoons of bee pollen grains. This should be thoroughly blended and applied with the fingertips. Leave it on for up to an hour. This cream should help to smooth out fine lines and correct dryness.

Propolis, honey and bee pollen have also been used successfully in the treatment of burns, gangrene, chicken pox (or any condition which involves itching and scarring of the skin) and wound healing.

Hayfever and Allergies

When you consider that such allergies as hayfever are actually caused by the body's oversensitivity to pollen, it must seem absurd to suggest that a possible treatment for the condition is pollen or honey, which contains pollen. Nevertheless, bee pollen has been found to be of benefit to sufferers by means of the process of desensitization (similar in action to acquiring immunity to certain diseases through inoculation), although it has to be admitted that scientific doubt has been cast on whether or not it is as effective as the hayfever injections administered by an allergist or doctor.

Hayfever is triggered by the body's overreaction to the particles of wind-borne pollen that are released by plants in the spring and early summer. Excessive amounts of histamine are produced and when it reaches the mucous membranes in the nose, they become inflamed and the result is a runny nose and breathing difficulties. Sinus headaches and earaches may also be experienced as the tissues in the sinuses swell, causing a build-up of pressure. If the person concerned has a tendency to asthma, the muscles around the bronchial tubes may contract, the tissues may swell and excess mucous may be secreted. It is important to treat allergies so that more serious problems do not develop.

Conventional treatment is to use antihistamines, which give temporary relief, antibiotics, where the allergy has progressed to an infection and hormones, such as cortisone. All of these have side-effects that may themselves be harmful. Bee pollen, however, if taken orally, can reduce the incidence of respiratory infections and allergic reactions without causing a reaction itself. One explanation is that the oesophagus and stomach quickly neutralize the allergens so that they do not produce an adverse reaction. Another possibility is that because some of the particles of bee pollen pass directly from the stomach into the bloodstream, without going through the normal process of digestion, desensitization takes place far more quickly.

One trial using bee pollen was carried out in Sweden in 1960 by Einar Helander, an allergist at Gothenburg. This involved 25 patients who were allergic to pollen, but who were otherwise healthy. When they were given a skin test of ground-up bee pollen tablets, they were found to be extremely allergic to them. When the same tablets and even larger doses, were taken orally, however, there was little allergic response.

Some natural therapists recommend taking natural honey, which contains bee pollen (a small amount on the tip of a spoon), for about six weeks before the beginning of the hayfever season. They have found that attacks are reduced in the first year and may be eliminated by the second year.

Propolis has also been found to be of benefit to allergy sufferers. It seems that the bioflavonoids in propolis help to block the leakage into the bloodstream of the excessive amounts of histamine that result in the allergic response. It has been found that some people develop a rash when taking propolis, although bee pollen is not known to have this effect.

There is anecdotal evidence that royal jelly has an anti-allergic effect. This may be because it contains bee pollen.

Radiation Therapy

There have been a few studies which have demonstrated that bee products may be of benefit to people undergoing radiation therapy.

In 1967, researchers William H. Shipman and Leonard J. Cole of the Life Science Division of the Stanford Research

Institute found that bee venom injected into mice helped to protect them from the effects of X-rays. They reasoned that melittin, which is found in bee venom, has a chemical structure similar to that of a detergent and may account for the slow absorption and spread of radiation in the body.

In 1973, Professor Osmanagic and others at the University Radiological Institute in Sarajevo conducted some trials with bee pollen and royal jelly capsules. Patients undergoing radiation therapy were experiencing adverse reactions in their blood, digestion, appetite and general wellbeing. X-rays affect the breakdown of proteins in the body so that excessive histamine is produced, which, in turn, produces symptoms of allergy. The initial test involved 16 women, whose symptoms ranged from tiredness and fainting to loss of weight, nausea and vomiting, liver damage and, in some, anaemia. It was found that the functioning of their livers greatly improved, with an increase in the production of glycogen, their red and white blood cell counts improved and their general condition improved, with many of their symptoms being reduced or entirely eliminated.

The same scientists then took three other groups of women. One group received the bee pollen and royal jelly capsules, one received a placebo and the last group were given nothing. The groups receiving the placebo or nothing showed a further deterioration in their health as a result of continued radiation treatment. Most of the women taking the bee pollen and royal jelly reported a 'good' to 'very good' improvement in their symptoms.

At the University of Vienna in Austria, Peter Hernuss conducted a study in which some of 25 women who had inoperative uterine cancer were undergoing radiation therapy and were suffering the symptoms of nausea, insomnia and general malaise. Of these women, 15 received a bee pollen supplement – 20 g three times a day. Those taking the supplement were found to be able to better tolerate the radiation treatment than the other 10, who received no bee pollen at all.

Other factors were also measured. The group taking bee pollen lost less vitamin C than did the other group; their blood levels of vitamin E increased; there was a 4 per cent increase in their red blood cells; their white blood cell count was up, as were their levels of albumin (a type of protein); cholesterol had reduced by 14 per cent. The authors thought that these beneficial effects of bee pollen were due to the increased levels of nutrients as well as the presence in bee pollen of beta-carotene, which is a free radical scavenger, scooping up the harmful free radicals released in the process of radiation (Hernuss, 1975).

There is some evidence that bee pollen may actually have an inhibitory effect on the growth of cancer cells and tumours. Royal jelly, too, may be of benefit to cancer sufferers. One paper written in Canada reported that ' ... the admixture of royal jelly with tumour cells before inoculation completely suppresses the development of transplantable mouse leukaemia and the formation of ascitic tumours in mice ... .This antitumour activity resides in the main fatty acid of royal jelly, 10-hydroxydecenoic acid ... .This effect was obtained only when the active material was mixed with the cancer cells prior to administration. Attempts to demonstrate protection after tumour implantation or by separate administration of royal jelly and leukaemia cells have as yet been unsuccessful. Further studies are in progress to determine whether the active material in royal jelly causes death of the tumour cells before inoculation ... ' (Townsend, Brown, Felauer and Hazlett, 1961).

Dr Osmanagic and his colleagues in Sarajevo also looked into whether or not propolis has anything to offer patients receiving radiation treatment. Over a period of two months, a group of such patients were given propolis, while another group were given a placebo. The results showed that the negative effects of radiation lessened or were even eliminated altogether by propolis. The other group could not report any improvements (Wade, *Propolis: Nature's Energizer*).

Prostatitis

Not only are bee products helpful for women at various stages in their lives, they are of particular benefit to the older man who may suffer from problems with his prostate gland. This gland is situated near the tube which exits from the male bladder and there may be times when it becomes enlarged, either by itself or because of an inflammation. An enlarged prostate gland can interfere with the excretion of urine so that the sufferer cannot empty his bladder entirely and may need to urinate frequently.

Where the condition is due to an inflammation (known as prostatitis), the symptoms may be as described and accompanied by pain. A number of studies have demonstrated that bee pollen can produce an improvement. Some of these go back to the early 1960s. One was conducted by three Swedish doctors (Drs Jonson, Leander and Professor Palmstierna), who found that out of 179 cases of persistent prostatitis, a bee pollen preparation, used in conjunction with orthodox measures, effected a 60 to 80 per cent improvement over another group of patients who received nothing but the usual treatments (Lyngheim and Scagnetti, *Bee Pollen: Nature's Miracle Health Food*).

In 1967, it was reported that one study in Uppsala involving 12 men found that 5 to 6 tablets taken first thing each day resulted in a dramatic improvement in 10 of the participants. The failure of the other two to respond was due to factors that negated the effect of the bee pollen.

Another trial led by urologists Alken, Jonsson and Rohl which took place at about the same time as the above found that 44 per cent of a group of 172 men suffering from prostatitis experienced relief after taking bee pollen.

These findings have been corroborated by research from Japan, undertaken by Dr Yutaka Saito of the Department of Urology at Nagasaki. He reported an 80 per cent cure rate (Lyngheim and Scagnetti, *Bee Pollen: Nature's miracle health food*).

A long-term study, which lasted three years, conducted by Professor Helse of the Urological Clinic of Magdeburg, resulted in not only the elimination of bacteria, but also an improvement in the mental health of those taking part and, in consequence, a beneficial effect on their marital relationships.

It is not entirely clear which elements of bee pollen are responsible for these results. One suggestion, based on the successful treatment of a group of prostatitis sufferers with zinc, is that it is the high levels of zinc in bee pollen that are responsible for this success. Also, it is recognized that a zinc deficiency can cause the prostate gland to enlarge and to malfunction. Zinc and, therefore, bee pollen are of particular benefit to those men whose prostate disorders are not caused by bacteria.

7

Safety, Interactions and Contraindications

Apart from the obvious question, answered in the previous chapter, as to whether or not bee pollen is a suitable treatment for hayfever sufferers, as with all treatments, it is necessary to ask whether or not there are any known side-effects from using bee products. Just because a substance is natural does not mean that it can never cause an adverse reaction.

Royal Jelly

Generally speaking, royal jelly is harmless for most people. If someone does suffer an allergic reaction after taking royal jelly, it may be that the allergy is triggered not by the jelly itself but by other ingredients within the product, such as wheatgerm oil, which would be a problem for coeliacs, for example.

Also, the reaction may not be attributable to the actual jelly but to the bee pollen grains it contains. Again, it is not possible to generalize as different people are allergic to different pollens. For example, in one study at the Mayo Clinic, three patients developed a severe response after consuming only one teaspoon, or less. It seems that they were, in fact, allergic to ragweed pollens (Cohen, *et al.*, 1979). Therefore, if you know you are allergic to certain pollens, it would be wise to test out the royal jelly first and even to check whether your digestive system can cope with it. Take only small amounts at first. If you start to suffer from a sore throat, a runny nose, or any other of the symptoms associated with pollen, you should reduce the amount you take to less than ⅛ teaspoon to see if the symptoms abate. If they persist, however, you should see your doctor.

Very rarely, royal jelly may contain a toxic pollen. Rhododendron, andromeda, corynocarpus, scolypoda, fagopyrum (only after drying), polygonum bistorta and hyoscayamus can have toxic effects.

Bee Pollen

In all of the studies cited in the earlier chapter about the benefits of bee pollen, no side-effects were recorded. Indeed, there is one known case of a man who was scared to give up his bee pollen because he had experienced a recurrence of his prostatitis when he had done so and therefore continued taking his supplements for nine years with no ill effect. However, the cautions outlined above apply even more obviously here. The same courses of action should be followed.

Honey

Raw, unprocessed honey contains pollen. Again, it does depend on the varieties of pollen contained in it as to whether there is likely to be an adverse reaction or not. For example, in India, the pollen from the *Lasiosiphon eriocephalus*, which was found in a honey, caused severe nausea and vomiting. Thus, the above comments concerning the other toxic pollens to avoid apply here, too.

Note also that honey should not be given to babies and young children as it has been known to cause infant botulism.

Propolis

Some authorities maintain that no adverse reactions to propolis have occurred. However, it has been suggested by others that propolis may bring a small number of people (between 1 in 2,000 and 5 per cent) out in a rash. This was confirmed by tests at the Edinburgh Royal Infirmary. However, those same people may exhibit no reaction when propolis is taken internally or as a gargle.

One way to test whether or not you are sensitive to it is to rub a little propolis on the side of your nose. If the skin reddens, you should avoid this product.

Interactions

Can you take bee products while using conventional medicines? The answer is yes as it does seem that they can actually *enhance* the actions of modern drugs. For example, propolis has been shown to facilitate the effects of antibiotics. It gives them a boost and helps them to work faster and more effectively. Furthermore, propolis can extend the shelf-life of antibiotic ointments from two to three months to nine to twelve months.

Bee pollen and royal jelly can help to neutralize some of the side-effects of conventional drug treatments and radiation therapy and can speed up the healing process. In some cases, people have found that they need to rely less on prescribed drugs, as with arthritis sufferers who have taken bee pollen.

There will, of course, always be sceptics and it is accepted that more scientific research needs to be carried out into the claims made for bee products. While waiting for scientific justification, though, you could be missing out on the very thing that will bring you relief for your condition. Honey and its companions have been around for thousands of years. Surely they are worth a try.

Bibliography

The Healing Power of Pollen with Propolis and Royal Jelly, Thorsons, 1989

HealthPlus, *NutriHealth Data*, 1994

Balch, James F., and Balch, Phyllis, A., *Prescription for Nutritional Healing*, Garden City Park, New York, Avery Publishing Group Inc., 1990

Brown, Royden, *Bee Hive Product Bible*, Garden City Park, New York, Avery Publishing Group Inc., 1993

Brown, R., *How to Live the Millennium: The bee pollen bible*, Hohm Press, 1994

Chaitow, Leon, *Amino Acids in Therapy*, Thorsons, 1985

Lyngheim, L., and Scagnetti, J., *Bee Pollen: Nature's miracle health food*, Melvin Powers Wilshire Book Company, 1979

Murray, Michael T., *Natural Alternatives to Over-the-Counter and Prescription Drugs*, New York, William Morrow and Co., Inc., 1994

Salaman, Maureen, and Scheer, James F., *Foods That Heal*, Menlo Park, California, M.K.S. Publishing, 1989

Stein, I., *Royal Jelly*, Thorsons, 1986

Wade, Carlson, *Propolis: Nature's energizer*, New Canaan, Connecticut, Keats Publishing Inc., 1983

Wade, Carlson, *Health from the Hive*, New Canaan, Connecticut, Keats Publishing Inc., 1992

Wade, Carlson, *Bee Pollen and Your Health*, Pirot Original Publishing, Connecticut, Keats Publishing Inc., 1992

References

Aagaard, K. Lund, *The Natural Product Propolis: The way to health*, Mentor, Denmark (1974) p. 21

Balalykina, V. P., *Propolis: Its antibacterial and therapeutic properties*, Kasan Publishing Co., USSR (1964)

Beck, Bodog F., *Bee Venom Therapy*, Bantam Books (1971)

Callais, Alain, 'Pollen – A Pharmaceutical Product', *L'Abeille de France et l'Apiculture*, 568, Paris, France (January, 1974)

Chauvin, R., 'Action sur les Mammiferes et sur Homme de la gelée royale', *L'Apiculteur*, Section Scientific, 101 Année, no. 4 (April, 1957)

Cohen, *et al.*, 'Acute allergic reaction after composite pollen ingestion', *Journal of Allergy and Clinical Immunology*, vol. 64, no. 4 (1979) pp. 270–4

Delperee, Robert, 'The Secrets of the Life of Bees', The Royal Society of the Naturalists of Mons, Belgium and Borinage, France, General Assembly, vol. XLIV, no.10 (1961)

Diamond, John, *BK – Behavioural Kinesiology*, (1978)

Gilliam, M., McCaughey, W. F., and Wintermute, B., 'Amino acids in pollens and nectars of citrus cultivars and in stored pollen and honey from honeybee colonies in citrus groves', *Journal of Apiculture Research*, vol. 19, no. 1 (1980) pp. 64–72

Hernuss, Peter, *et al.*, 'Pollen Diet as an Adjunct of Radiation Therapy in Gynecological Carcinomas', Strahleutherapic (1975)

Jorde, W., and Linskens, H. F., *German Acta Allergol*, vol. 29 (1974) pp. 165–70

Lunden, R., 'A short introduction to the literature on pollen chemistry', vol. 66 (1954) pp. 201–13

Osmanagic, I., 'Clinical Testing of Melbrosia on Women Suffering from Climacteric Syndrome', Endocrinological Department of the University Clinic for Women, Medical Faculty, Sarajevo, Yugoslavia (May 1972)

Perivale, Lloyd, *American Bee Journal* (1955)

Pokrajcic, L., and Osmanagic, I., 'Treatment with Melbrosia of Dysmenorrhoea in Adolescence', Endocrinological Department of the University Clinic for Women, Medical Faculty, Sarajevo, Yugoslavia (March, 1976)

Saenz, A., 'Biology, Biochemistry and the Therapeutic Effects of Royal Jelly in Human Pathology', Pasteur Institute, Paris, France (July, 1984)

Taranov, I., Institute of Apiculture, USSR (1977)

Townsend, G. F., Brown, W. H., Felauer, E. E., Hazlett, B., Departments of Apiculture and Chemistry, Ontario Agricultural College, Guelph, Ontario, and Department of Therapeutics, University of Toronto, Toronto, Ontario, 'Studies on the In Vitro Antitumour Activity from Royal Jelly Against Transplantable Mouse Leukemia', *Canadian Journal of Biochemistry and Physiology*, vol. 36 (1961)

Vinogradova, T. V., and Zajceva, G. P., *American Chiropractor*, vol.2, no.2, (February, 1979)

Index

Of further interest...

Nutrients for Health:
Green-Lipped Mussel

HELPING IN THE TREATMENT OF OSTEO-
AND RHEUMATOID ARTHRITIS

John E. Croft

All known minerals are contained in the sea and the shell-fish that live there concentrate within their system a unique 'cocktail' of trace elements. An extract from one such shell-fish, the New Zealand green-lipped mussel, has been found to relieve symptoms of osteo- and rheumatoid arthritis. Revised and updated, this book is about the green-lipped mussel and the safe and effective treatment that has been developed from it, a treatment which offers freedom from pain and a restoration of mobility for many sufferers of arthritis.

Nutrients for Health:
Blue-Green Algae

THE 'SUPERFOOD' FOR HEALTH AND WELL-BEING

Paul Smith

Blue-green algae has been harvested for hundreds of years. In the past decde it has been recognized by scientists as a rich source of food, containing an almost perfect balance of nutrients.

Blue-green algae is currently catching the attention of the world's media with claims that it boosts energy, improves sleep, reduces allergies, migraines, stress and PMT, and strengthens the body's immune system. In the United States it is now a multi-million pound industry and is hailed as Hollywood's new favourite supplement.

Paul Smith provides an accessible, readable and authoritative general introduction to this nutritious 'superfood'.

Nutrients for Health:
Evening Primrose Oil

BORAGE OIL, BLACKCURRANT OIL
AND OTHER RICH SOURCES OF GLA

Hasnain Walji

Evening primrose oil is high in the rare gammalinolenic acid (GLA) and is a rich source of essential fatty acids which are fundamental for good health.

The success of evening primrose oil over the last decade has been phenomenal. It is one of the most popular products sold in health food stores and it can now be classified as a drug, prescribed regularly by doctors for a wide range of conditions.

This accessible and authoritative book explains how evening primrose oil – and other oils rich in GLA – can play an important role in maintaining healthy skin, hormonal balance and supple joints.

Nutrients for Health:
Folic Acid

ESSENTIAL DURING PREGNANCY
AND FOR HEALTHY LIVING

Hasnain Walji

Folic acid is essential for the formation of red blood cells and growth. Today, its vital role in health is beyond dispute.

Pregnant women are the most important group of people that need folic acid. Scientific research has proved beyond doubt that it can prevent neural tube defects such as spina bifida and the government has launched a campaign to encourage women of child-bearing age to increase their daily intake.

Yet the general public is often either unaware, confused or simply ignorant of the health benefits of folic acid. In this easy-to-read book, Hasnain Walji explains clearly how important it is for pregnant women and young children – and how we can all benefit from this 'rising star' in the world of nutrition.

NUTRIENTS FOR HEALTH:		
GREEN-LIPPED MUSSEL	0 7225 3171 0	£3.99
NUTRIENTS FOR HEALTH:		
BLUE-GREEN ALGAE	0 7225 3319 5	£3.99
NUTRIENTS FOR HEALTH:		
EVENING PRIMROSE OIL	0 7225 3324 1	£3.99
NUTRIENTS FOR HEALTH:		
FOLIC ACID	0 7225 3320 9	£3.99

All these books are available from your local bookseller or can be ordered direct from the publishers.

To order direct just tick the titles you want and fill in the form below:

Name: ....

Address: ....

....

.... Postcode....................................

Send to Thorsons Mail Order, Dept 3, HarperCollins*Publishers*, Westerhill Road, Bishopbriggs, Glasgow G64 2QT.

Please enclose a cheque or postal order or your authority to debit your Visa/Access account –

Credit card no: ....

Expiry date: ....

Signature: ....

– up to the value of the cover price plus:
UK & BFPO: Add £1.00 for the first book and 25p for each additional book ordered.
Overseas orders including Eire: Please add £2.95 service charge. Books will be sent by surface mail but quotes for airmail dispatches will be given on request.

24-HOUR TELEPHONE ORDERING SERVICE FOR ACCESS/VISA CARDHOLDERS — TEL: 0141 772 2281.